# The Tyranny of

CW00519787

# 50 Years of '
# 'Change' in the NHS; the unforeseen consequences, accumulation of clutter, nonsense and Strikes!

## ALLOWING THE NHS TO BECOME 'HUMAN' AGAIN

The dynamics that have been allowed to develop within the Behemoth that the NHS has become are destroying it.

The basics of health care as in the early years of the NHS need to be returned to when doctors were listened to and felt that they were responsible for and in consequence proud of the nation's health system.

The prescription needed for this to happen is for the Health Secretary, currently Mr Jeremy Hunt to ask the medics for their examples of where money is being used in ways that don't help them look after their patients.This would start the conversation that is needed to restore the NHS to a time when the people on the ground mattered, that is listened to, and when in consequence health care in the UK was also much more efficient as well as more human and therefore more humane for both patients and staff

About the author

Dr Rod Storring is a consultant physician.
His experience of the NHS totals more than 50 years,
initially as a medical student, then as a junior doctor
progressing to become a consultant in a University District
General Hospital. Finally he became a consultant
physician in the community.

His other book is 'A Doctor's Life'

Email address, r.storring@hotmail.com

**Amazon publication**

**FOREWORD**

The authority for these writings is drawn from my experience of more than 50 years as a medical doctor working in the NHS, the major part as a Consultant Physician in a University District General Hospital and then as a Respiratory Consultant Physician in the Community.

My reasons for these writings are threefold.

Firstly it is to provide historical explanations for the dysfunctional and impersonal mess that the NHS has got itself into.

Secondly to help the current debate of, 'more funding is needed' against the notion that this would be 'throwing good money after bad'

Thirdly to suggest a way for the NHS to return to a more efficient and less costly health care system

**Shortened extracts from comments on 'Tyranny'**

-Thanks for allowing me to see this excellent manuscript. I think that there is a huge amount here which clearly needs to be said

-I very much enjoyed reading your book on the future of the NHS. I have not seen a discussion on the matter that so comprehensively covers areas that many do not seem willing to broach.
I thought your ideas were spot on

- I think it is an excellent summary of both the problems and solutions within our current NHS

-We have lost the relationships between junior doctors, consultants and nurses exactly in the way that you describe and this has led to alienated professionals trying to look after alienated patients in an alienated system

-Turning to solutions, I entirely agree that "the money should flow from what arises out of the doctor/patient encounter and be seen to do so". This can be achieved through your model of "The details of how this is to be carried out and funded needing medical supervision".

## Acknowledgements

I would like to thank an old school friend Dr Chris Gardner-Thorpe for his major efforts with editing and added to this, his encouragement.Others I would like to thank for suggestions and support are my brother, Patrick; my son David and partner Jay; my daughter Nicola in training to be a paediatrician; my neighbour Joe Stuckey, recently in NHS IT; friends,Philip Bedford and Dr John Glees; Angela, previous ward sister; Cilla, medical secretary;Suba Biggs clinical audit administrator;John Bald whose experiences in the education system in the UK are not too dissimilar to mine in the NHS system.

To those I have not mentioned I apologise and add that what I have written is also very dependent on my experiences with the patients I have seen over the years and the colleagues I have worked with.

# THE TYRANNY OF A SYSTEM - THE NHS

# CONTENTS

# INTRODUCTION

In today's never ending discussions about Britain's National Health Service (NHS) the recurring questions are - should it survive? and, can it? Recently a consultant surgeon was reported in The London Times as saying, "I don't matter any more than the ward cleaner". The shameful truth is that the ward cleaner does not matter either. This would not have been the case until recent years.The unprecedented walkout by junior doctors is a result of the blatant disregard for the profession. The only way to 'matter' is to strike.From 1997 to 2012 health expenditure in the NHS increased by 373%. This massive extra funding did not result in proportionate health gains. Would this have been different in a system where individuals still mattered, and where individuals were not being tyrannised by the system,- the NHS? The purpose of this publication is to record many of the changes in the NHS that I experienced over a period of 50 years, initially as a medical student and then as a doctor.The consequences of these changes described are mostly unforeseen, inevitable in a complex system. The result is an NHS which most doctors do not believe can survive for very much longer.It is the author's thesis that the 'clutter and nonsense' have got in the way of the highly trained health care professionals who look after the patients.

The question is, if the NHS went back to its early years with patient needs at the forefront, would efficiency increase, costs go down and staff satisfaction and patient outcomes improve? The author's belief is that if people working in the NHS started to matter again and if once more the organisation was allowed to become 'human' in the way it used to be, the calls for its abandonment would cease.The author's further belief is that the changes necessary to bring this about will need a group or groups of doctors to run with the ideas proposed in chapter 12 and in part three of this publication.What is needed is a bottom-up approach though expert non-medical help will be needed by the medics. It would surprise the author if political support did not materialise. Were the current Secretary of State for Health, Jeremy Hunt at the forefront of that, he might even be remembered fondly by the medical profession and the nation.

This publication is divided into three parts.

The first part deals with the NHS from 1948 to the present and describes how The NHS has developed in virtue of its ingredients, actual and ideological which, as time has passed, have got in the way, to a greater or lesser extent to the provision of satisfactory health care for the nation.Also described are the changes and ideas introduced into the NHS which have had significant, unforeseen and damaging consequences.

The second part consists of short accounts of some of the changes and ideas that have been added to the NHS over the year together with their negative consequences and what can be done about them?

In part three,-'The Way Forward',my suggestion is that to repair the damage that has accumulated in the NHS over the years, the NHS needs a 'return to the future' , namely to go back to the basics of health care which dominated what happened in the NHS in its early years. Everything that at the moment is getting in the way of doctors discharging their responsibilities to their patients needs to be removed.Inadequate funding held back the development of the NHS in former years and should not have been tolerated by the medical profession. This time the funding will have to be more appropriate than previously but, most important, has to be supervised by the front-line clinicians.

Of particular interest at the moment is that the USA is looking at the possibility of adopting a single-payer health service which for the most part is provided in the UK by the NHS. American doctors are as fed up as their British counterparts but for very different reasons. Their health system is dominated by a multi-billion dollar medical insurance industry. There are numerous obstacles and difficulties that the US doctor has to negotiate in this system and these interfere with patient care, hence their interest in the NHS and of their worries about its shortcomings which as this book demonstrates are actually the result of the mess that we have made of it rather than the necessary result of a single- payer health service.

**PART ONE**

**The NHS, 1948 to the present.**

The main reason for the creation of the NHS was that previously many people were denied health care because they were poor. A poster published in July 1948 informed the population of the purpose of the NHS - 'it will relieve your money worries in times of illness'.

However with a socialist mandate and given the socially divisive pre-war period it made sense for the Attlee Government to establish and maintain national social cohesion in the victorious one-nation post-war Britain and, so far as health was concerned, it was decided that not only will everyone be able to access medical care but that this care would also be free. However, leaving aside the politics, making it free for everyone was unnecessary as in fact only the poor needed help to access health care. The human right that should have been aimed at was to make certain that everyone should have access to affordable care. In the event though, providing free health care for everyone in Britain by the creation of the NHS was achieved to a great extent in the early decades of the NHS. Unfortunately at present there are again many who cannot afford adequate medical care which in many parts of the UK, particularly in the cities, is frequently only available to those who can afford to pay for it.

Central to the NHS, and in the past seen worldwide as the 'jewel in the crown' of the NHS, is General Practice. Continuity of care, seeing the same doctor at each visit, knowing and being known by the doctor, having enough time with the doctor and having ready access to the doctor, all of which are seen by many as essential for patient care, is disappearing very rapidly from General Practice in the NHS.

Contrast our health care with the rest of Western Europe. Despite the absence of an NHS in other countries, Western Europeans on the continent are not denied medical care on grounds of inability to pay and, in terms of many patient outcomes, often seem to do be getting better medical care than is available in the UK.

Given that the reason for the creation of the NHS appears to have been lost sight of, do we still need the NHS? Should we be looking for an alternative to the NHS as a way of continuing to provide us with health care? and should it continue to be for the most part free? Instead of doing away with the NHS however, perhaps something can be done that would restore it as a free-for-all health service for everyone entitled to it. As mentioned previously, emotionally this would be more satisfying to a nation that still sees the NHS as embodying the values of its nationhood as they existed in the immediate post-war period. As an aside, some have pointed out that the NHS is treated by the media, the politicians and the public, and arguably to the disadvantage of health care in the UK, as a quasi-national religion, a 'Sacred Cow'. Unfortunately this can get in the way of rational thought and the sensible thing may be to break this linking of health care and nationhood as envisaged in the immediate post-war period.

In the light of current thinking we can not be optimistic that 'mending' the NHS is achievable and over the years there have been many vain attempts to put it right. There is however a possibility of improving the NHS and therefore retaining the NHS when examining the changes that have happened in the NHS and which have over the last 50 years resulted in the complex and often dysfunctional health care system we now have in the UK. If we did that, there would then be the possibility of seeing a way to return to the basics of patient care that existed in the early decades of the NHS but which to many patients, doctors, nurses and other healthcare workers alike have been lost sight of in the current NHS.

Of course everything wasn't perfect in those early decades. Unfortunately during those early years the NHS was underfunded and the medical leaders of those years must bear some responsibility for that – they should have insisted on adequate funding but instead the leaders of the profession allowed the politicians to get away with the chronic underfunding of health care in the UK and in consequence patient care in the UK lagged behind the rest of Western Europe. With the NHS in trouble at the moment there is little chance of catching up this lost ground unless there is a radical re-think.

As a complex system, the introduction of any changes and new ideas in the NHS will result in consequences often unforeseen. Needless to say, with the increasing number of failures in the NHS these changes and new ideas, and therefore their consequences, have been numerous and accelerating in recent years. Many of these consequences have been and continue to be toxic to the system.

The purpose of this publication is to start a critical and constructive examination of the NHS in relation to some of the significant changes and ideas together with their consequences that have occurred during the nearly half century of my time in the NHS, initially as a medical student and then as a doctor.

Also included are some of the scene-setting ingredients that were already there when I started in 1960 such as equity and feelings of nationhood. At different times these have distorted the basics needed for providing adequate health care for a population.

Now acknowledged as a major distorting factor for the provision of efficient health care has been the increasing central control exerted by Whitehall in recent decades. The idea that presaged top down management of the NHS was of course expressed in Aneurin Bevan's notorious promise that 'if a bedpan dropped in a hospital corridor, the reverberations should echo in Whitehall'.

Over the years there have also been many societal changes and not surprisingly and to a variable extent some of these have made their way into the society and societies that make up the NHS. Where these have made a difference to the NHS is also important, and with that the question arises as to whether these societal changes might have been looked at more closely before incorporating them into the NHS.

An example is the loss of hierarchy and with it the loss of the structure which inevitably accompanies a hierarchy. Linked to this is equity.The Socialist Health Association whose progenitor, the Socialist Medical Association, started in 1930 within the Labour Party, still has as its purpose - 'greater commitment to the real purpose of the NHS – equity'. What is often forgotten when decisions have to be made is that equity, although a value, can and should be trumped when appropriate. This is unlikely to happen though if the Socialist Health Association or any like minded folk are deciding what to do.

Another example is linked to trying to achieve gender equality. As it happens, females aged 18 are better than males at taking A levels and continuing to use this as a measure for entrance to a medical training has resulted in some medical schools admitting up to 70% female students.The result is a large increase in female doctors and in consequence an increasing proportion of doctors perfectly happy to work part-time. One result of this is fragmented patient care particularly in general practice as mentioned already. There are other examples of unforeseen consequences.(see chapter eight)

Given the complexities of what is now the NHS, a reminder of the basics of health care is needed. In the early decades of the NHS, these basics were central to what was going on in the UK both in General Practice and in the hospitals. Doctors were able to treat patients and take responsibility for them as they felt their training, experience and peer opinion permitted.

In a profession as old as the medical one, the opinions of peers are immensely powerful. Doctors like everyone else find that embarrassment is one of the most powerful of forces. Doctors do not like making mistakes. Doctors do not require the tick-boxing tyranny, post-Shipman scrutiny and the lack of trust implicit in the hoops through which they now have to jump in their daily work. Basic medical care needs to be returned to. It should not be frustrated by the mistrust that is implied in the many ways that Whitehall is trying to control what is happening at the level of patient-care.

Examples of what it is still possible for doctors to do medically can be seen particularly in the cities where private medicine is flourishing and especially in primary care. Here GPs know their patients, provide continuity of care that can be excellent as well as efficient and, of course, are unencumbered by the bureaucracy of the NHS.

Since managers have replaced administrators in the NHS in the last 25 years, the possibility of this sort of medical practice has been ignored increasingly. The result has been the loss of the good will of the medical profession as well as their ability to look after their patients as they used to be able to do. The irony is that this change from 'administrator' to 'manager' was merely a re-naming of the NHS administrator.What's in a name?

There is a big difference in the meaning of the words 'administrator' and 'manager'. An administrator administers. Before 'the age of management' in the NHS, to administer meant administering the provision of the support needed for patient care. To be a manager suggests a position rather higher in the organisation than that of an administrator and certainly denotes a different relationship to doctors who should have remained in charge of the essentials as to what has to be done for patients. Doctors no longer feel in charge in the way that they did and in the way they feel is still necessary.

The major change though was that these managers were now part of government policies to increase the efficiency of public service. The name given to this movement was 'Public Service Management' which introduced the three Ms - markets, management and measurement. The idea was to introduce efficiencies that were thought to be more accessible using ideas to do with the market place. However, the three Ms each have unforeseen and negative consequences. After decades of underfunding. the government at last recognised that the important reason for the inadequacies of the NHS was underfunding, and this was rectified to some extent in the early 2000s.

Surprisingly, patient outcomes did not improve as a result of the massive amount of money poured into the NHS.(From 1997 to 2012 there was an increase of 373%, approximately, £100 billion in funding).

Were the three Ms, now in place, anything to do with that failure? Would the result of this extra funding have been different if the doctors and previous administrators were still running the show?Doctors have little doubt that the NHS would now be in much better shape if that had been the case.

The difference between the two scenarios is that with the three Ms the basics of health care, as outlined above, has held less and less importance in the NHS. Doctors who are fundamental to treating patients now feel themselves disempowered and tyrannised by the system within which they are trying to treat their patients. Needless to say their job satisfaction suffers , as does patient care.

This relationship between both how well a doctor feels able to look after patients and patient satisfaction seems intuitively obvious but is also demonstrated in the annual staff satisfaction surveys held throughout the NHS when these are looked at in relation to patient outcomes. The answer to one of the questions in the questionnaire, 'Are you able to do your job to a standard you are pleased with?', distinguishes very clearly between poorly and well performing Trusts. Aiming for a satisfactory answer to this question within a Trust would be a very much more successful target than many of the other targets imposed by Whitehall over the years. The reason for this being so is that motivated doctors are essential for excellent health care.

To achieve both of these it is necessary to look for reasons why the NHS has gone wrong. This is what part two is about.

(As a footnote, each chapter in part two is comprehensive to its subject matter. However because of the interconnectedness of the many parts of the NHS, some repetition chapter to chapter is inevitable)

**Part Two**

**How the NHS has gone wrong**

**Chapter One**

**Hierarchy, patient care and the NHS**


Society 50 years ago was much more hierarchical than it is now.This is also true for the NHS. Is this loss in hierarchical structure in the NHS important and does it explain in any way the troubles of today's NHS? Around what was the hierarchical structure of the NHS arranged in 1960 when I became a medical student?Are the criteria that underpinned this hierarchical structure at that time still valid to some extent in today's world?

So far as Western Civilisation is concerned the notion of hierarchy, as also the word, originated in a religious setting in Ancient Greece where at the top of the hierarchy was the high priest and leader of the sacred rights. Things were of course very different by the time I started my time in the NHS in 1960, although still recognisable as 'high priests' and 'leaders of the sacred rights', were doctors, particularly the consultants.

That this picture can amuse us and even seem ridiculous 50 years later probably says more about us now, than indicate that there was something wrong with how things were.

Where, if anywhere, has the power, energy and authority that those doctors needed to drive what was happening in the NHS in those days gone? The fact is that with the withdrawal of all of this from the doctors, no one else appears any longer to have a grip on what is happening. Individuals from Ministers of Health to Trust CEOs and lesser individuals in the NHS get blamed and sacked from time to time, but how responsible were they for what they were sacked for,-probably not much.

The idea of a national health service continues to seduce us into continuing to attribute to it the power and authority to look after our health needs, but unfortunately the reality is that what was created in 1948 and worked well, though markedly underfunded over the initial decades, has morphed into 'The NHS' which now has many of the characteristics of a 'Sacred Cow'.

The strong belief system required for the survival of this particular 'Holy Cow' is weakening as we fall behind health care systems in other countries, experience the growing inefficiencies and inadequacies of the NHS and end up wondering where all the tax payer's money is going and asking the question whether the NHS is still worth it.

In the early decades of the NHS when an obvious hierarchy was still in place, the underfunding of the service was a major problem for providing an adequate health service for the country.Unfortunately proper funding had to wait until the time when doctors were no longer being listened to.The earlier hierarchy with doctors appearing to run the show certainly at the clinical level, had been lost.The chances are that had the money arrived earlier, we would now have an NHS that would in deed be a world beater.

What were the pluses and minuses of this earlier hierarchy?What was its history? How much of that history was to do with what was, and in reality is still required for running a health service, and how much was it to do with the unfairnesses in the society of those times?

A discussion on hierarchy in the UK is inseparable from our feelings about class although almost certainly none of these instincts will be mentioned. Class is a national obsession though almost always as sub-text and therefore usually not acknowledged as a cause of possible bias.

Over the 50 years in question society has also become more socialistic. A colleague brought up in what was then Yugoslavia even goes so far as to to say that living in Britain now is more communistic than life ever was behind the Iron Curtain. He was referring to the control over the individual that has been increasing inexorably in the UK. but also to the egalitarianism that has become exaggerated beyond what a fair-minded and flourishing community actually requires and is good for it.Individuals have to a large extent been written out of today's narrative which nowadays tends to be about teams.

Mention tick boxes, form filling, guidelines, health and safety, managers monitoring targets and the decisions of the endless number of committees of today's NHS, human resource departments, etc to a doctor struggling to deal with the basics of patient care on a daily basis and listen to the lack of freedom and resulting lack of enjoyment from work available for today's doctor.

'The good days of the NHS have gone' is the usual comment from the doctors retiring long before reaching the age at which their predecessors had given up doctoring. By the 'good days' the reference for the most part is to a previous time when the doctor had been able freely as a professional to do the best for the patient using the knowledge, experience and expertise that had been acquired over the years.

So far as the 'exaggerated egalitarianism' referred to above, the modern doctor is now seen merely as belonging to one of the numerous health care professional groups each with their hierarchies, rules, regulations and voice in the NHS.In this arrangement it isn't difficult to see how medical professionalism isn't taken seriously enough.

The hierarchy that was in place in my teaching hospital in 1960 was to an important extent arranged around what the hospital was for, that is looking after the patients who came through the door whilst teaching their 'apprentices', medical students and junior doctors how this is done.This arrangement had developed naturally over the years since the hospital's beginning in the 18th century and was for the most part harmonious and effective. The fact that some of the consultants mistook their position in this hierarchy as personal to them and behaved accordingly was a shame but not a necessary accompaniment to the hierarchical structure that was in place.

That the consultants occupied the top of the hierarchy made sense for many reasons the main one being that the basics of what the whole business was about was under the control of the most highly trained group in the hospital who saw to it whilst working effectively with their nurse colleagues, that the best was done for the patients.

The distractions from these basics which have built up over the last 50 years are what this publication is about. These distractions which get in the way of the doctor-patient relationship have to be removed in order to restore the NHS into an effective way of looking after the sick.

The sick will always be with us however effective public health measures are and it is through the perspective of folk needing medical attention that the NHS will always be seen.

If pivotal to this is the doctor-patient relationship, then anything else that NHS money is to be spent on has to stem from this and its needs, and be seen to do so.Inevitably this will restore what the hierarchical structure was about.

My hope is that the doctors of that future will deal with it rather better than their predecessors did.

The results of restoring 'what the hierarchical structure was about' will be a much improved as well as a more cost effective NHS.

**Chapter Two**

## QUALITY AND OUTCOMES FRAMEWORK (QOF)

Definition of the word bribe:-something valuable (such as money) that is given in order to get someone to do something (Merriam Webster).

The Quality and Outcomes Framework (QOF) is a system for the performance management and payment of general practitioners (GPs) in the National Health Service. QOF money amounts to about a third of a GP's income and is their only way of increasing that income. It was introduced as part of the new general medical services (GMS) contract in April 2004 as agreed to by the British Medical Association (BMA)The QOF rewards GPs for implementing 'good practice' in their surgeries.'Good practice' as mentioned here ought to be the professional duty of doctors.That it seemed necessary to bribe them, 'bribed' as defined above, to perform as they should, ought to have been seen by doctors as unacceptable. There must be other ways for a profession to make sure that the members of that profession behave as they should without having to bribe them.

That it was accepted by their professional body, the BMA says a lot about the BMA. Unfortunately the BMA frequently appears to be more interested in maximising its doctors' incomes than protecting its doctors' professionalism. There are other examples of the BMA behaving similarly.Ultimately this sort of behaviour results in poorer patient care.

What are the results of introducing the QOF system?

QOF income is generated by accumulating QOF points. This consists of ticking boxes. When ticking boxes generates income it is only human for this activity to become rather important for the individual doctor. Unfortunately this results in unforeseen and unfortunate consequences.

-Good practice that the QOF system doesn't recognise, like listening to the patient, become less important.

-Listening to the patient and talking to them is also impeded by the system within which QOF operates.

-In the modern GP surgery there are now three agents present, the patient, the doctor and the computer.For various reasons the last, the computer gets in the way of the doctor-patient consultation where only two agents should be present.

-In which ways is the computer an agent?The computer records, and now with increasing frequency dictates what the doctor should and shouldn't do. This is an important cause of the loss of clinical freedom of GPs.

-QOF points are accumulated by what the doctor feeds into the computer.The patient comes into the surgery with a problem. The doctor checks on the computer where QOF points can be gained and not infrequently will then ask QOF-directed questions that have nothing to do with what is troubling the patient.The patient is unaware of this other activity going on as the GP earns another fiver here and a tenner there. With the consultation limited to ten minutes (see reference to 'Ten minute consultations' in chapter 10) and the distractions provided by earning QOF money, is it surprising that the matter that should be in hand, ie dealing with the patient's problem, is likely to have been undermined?

-Many QOF points are linked to following the national guidelines.But as in my chapter on guidelines these have significant downsides and are of overall questionable benefit.

-My personal experience came about when I became a consultant community chest physician.Part of the purpose of this post was to educate the GPs in chest medicine. After some time I came to the conclusion that I was beating my head against a brick wall so far as educating the GPs was concerned. For the most part they had handed the care of the chest patients to their nurses to guideline-manage and collect the relevant QOF points.

# Chapter Three

## The 2003 GP contract and 'Fools Gold'

In 1948 Aneurin Bevan 'stuffed the mouths of hospital consultants with gold' and thereby succeeded in getting the NHS started. In contrast the gold in the 2003 GP contract has turned out to be 'fools gold' for GPs, their patients and the NHS.

The GPs on the BMA negotiating team should have been alerted by their reactions, of being 'shocked' and 'stunned', to what the government agreed to. Their instincts as doctors and GPs should have persuaded them not to be greedy in view of the fact that important aspects of the professionalism to do with being a GP were being sacrificed by agreeing to that contract.The consequences are now coming home to roost.

GPs are stressed, unhappy, job satisfaction is poor, GPs are retiring early and recruitment is much lower than it used to be.

The large extra payments for GPs in that contract was dealt with in the last chapter.'QOF' money was in part to get all GPs to deliver the health care that the good GPs were already giving their patients.That a group of professionals needed to be paid more to get them do their job properly is bad enough, but that this was then to be delivered by ticking boxes had to be wrong and has contributed to the poor morale in General Practice.

In addition the government allowed the GPs to opt out of out-of-hours only asking for a 6% cut in pay.One doctor on the negotiating committee commented, 'We got rid of it for effectively 6% of the value of the contract. It was just stunning. Nobody in my position had ever believed we could pull it off but to get it for 6% was a bit of a laugh.'

What are the negative and unexpected consequences of the 2003 GP contract?

-The undermining of the GP partner system where patients know who their GP is, don't see a different GP on each visit and where the family doctor/friend used to be common and where an individual doctor took responsibility for individual patients. Continuity of care is an essential in patient care and nowadays appears to be more and more difficult to deliver.

-QOF income is considerable and given the availability of trained GPs who can be hired as locum, salaried and part-time GPs, why share that income by taking on a new partner?Does this built-in disincentive to appoint GP partners explain why their numbers are going down. In addition, and sadly the youngsters are having difficulties in getting a partnership unless there is a family connection!

-On the other hand, GPs are opting out of partnership because of all the bureaucracy involved, preferring to do be a GP locum instead.

-'I never see the same GP twice', 'I don't know who my GP is' are experiences common to the UK patient.
-ticking boxes gets in the way of listening to the patient which also gets in the way of job satisfaction as well as 'proper doctoring'.

-There are some practices where mutual doctor/patient mistrust is marked. This results in poor patient care as well as loss of patient cooperation together with the loss of control of the practice that the GPs had in the past.
-25% reduction of the number of patients on practice lists.Patients are now having difficulties getting on to a GP list.
-there are now three agencies in the consulting room, the GP, the patient and the computer? The importance of needing to satisfy the last is getting in the way of the doctor-patient relationship.

The question is how to undo the damage done by the 2003 contract.

A new GP contract is required and this has to remember three basic facts.

1) General Practice provided the strength of the NHS. Being a family doctor was the career fulfilment for so many general practitioners in the past

2) The standards of good medical practice should be regulated by the profession and therefore should not have to be bought by the government as a top-up

income (QOF) earned by hitting targets under a performance-related bonus scheme.

3) The GPs need again to be in charge and responsible for their patients 24/7. Years ago, also by cooperating with neighbouring practices, many of them were able to provide this efficiently and well. They managed to off-load this responsibility for minimal loss of income in 2003.

The money needed to pay the GPs again for this, would be available, firstly, by diverting the top-up income(QOF), secondly, a lot of money would be available with the dramatic reduction in A/E and hospital patient numbers that will inevitably follow the GPs again being in charge of their patients. Third, from the money that will no longer be needed to cover off-duty GPs. As it is this cover excites much negative media comment.

**Chapter Four**

**'Nurses are not doctors' hand maidens'**

Many years ago the statement that heads this section was probably said as a joke. Unfortunately in more recent times decades of trainee nurses have had this repeatedly told them by their nursing tutors. It has become a mantra in the Nursing Profession. Given that doctors and nurses need to work well together to achieve best patient care, has this notion and the thinking around it, and taken as seriously as it has been by the nursing profession, had a damaging effect on patient care in the UK?It would be surprising if it hadn't!

In recent years explanations have been looked for to explain poor nursing and lack of compassion amongst nurses.

Nurses of previous years now in later life, have been known to be 'appalled' at the modern standard of nursing when they now experience it as patients. The one explanation for poor nursing that I have not seen given, and in my judgement is hugely important, is that doctors and nurses no longer work together in the way that they used to. A distinct separation has taken place.

Nurses now see themselves as in a health care profession governed by its own disciplines, tasks, rules and regulations very much as they see doctors in another, but separate body of health care professionals. So far as the nurses are concerned the two groups are doing something entirely separate to the patients.As a result the nurses are now self-evidently no one's 'handmaiden'.

The term 'handmaiden' as well as having a serving meaning, also has a meaning to do with status, here of course in relation to doctors. Is the introduction of the need for nurses to have degrees an accident? Is it any accident that we now have 'nurse-consultants' and 'nurse-specialists'? As it happens, these titles and roles have emerged in part as a result of the introduction of guidelines which in turn have considerable downsides and are of questionable overall value (see guidelines).

Has the idea of developing nurses as a separate health care professional group independent of doctors, led to poorer care of patients? Has it reduced the job satisfaction of nurses? The result of the nurse/doctor separation has resulted in the loss of the doctor-nurse teamwork that used to exist. This is coupled with nurses being seen as un-necessarily unhelpful to doctors.Inevitably both of these have been to the detriment of patient care.

The reasons for this doctor/nurse separation are many but it is not difficult to see the connections between the 'handmaiden' reference, late 20th century feminism and the psychological motivation behind nursing leaders wanting to strengthen the status as they see it of the nursing profession. (In relation to feminism, it is ironical that female doctors will in the not too distant future, be in the majority in the UK).

This separation, nurses from doctors has been brought about in many ways.Nurse training used to be done in hospitals with the clinical lectures given by the medical staff working in those hospitals. As a result, nurses and doctors had a common language and understanding about what was wrong with the patients that they were both looking after in the wards. All too frequently this common understanding of what is going on is no longer there. Trainee nurses are now taught about diseases in college by Nurse Lecturers.These lecturers used to be clinical nurses, often a long time ago. Their knowledge of diseases cannot be comparable to that of the experienced physicians and surgeons who used to teach the nurses of previous generations.

Another example of the nurses going their own way is to do with the nursing record previously known as the 'Kardex'. This used to provide a good account of what was happening to the patient. This nursing record allowed useful information for nurses and doctors to share in the care of their patients.

Nurse leaders then introduced the Nursing Process which was designed to help to evaluate in a systematic way what nurses did. This was linked to the idea of the need to establish measurables as it were for the Nursing Profession to demonstrate itself as more objective and therefore in a sense scientific. Unfortunately the consequence was the loss of the narrative in the nursing record.What replaced it was a list of actual and possible 'nursing problems' that a patient had and which needed nursing attention.this was called a 'problem orientated nursing record'. As a result of the loss of the patient narrative, no one, neither doctors nor nurses were then in a position to know from the nursing record what had been happening to the patient! This was particularly troublesome for the doctors as they are not usually permanently in the ward, and therefore need information about patients from the ward nurses looking after these patients.

There are many other examples where this separation of the nurse's and doctor's roles in patient care have occurred but a very telling example is to do with national clinical guidelines that have been introduced in recent years.

What is particularly interesting when looking at 'unexpected consequences' in the 'complex system' that is the NHS, is that with this example the consequences are so widespread (also see section on guidelines).

The consequences of what is seen as the over-specialisation of medical care which has developed in recent years, will be dealt with later.In the context though of guidelines, specialists develop these for non-specialists, including nurses to follow and here the role of the nurse becomes interesting and to some extent worrying.

Working with guidelines and how they now function in the NHS, a nurse training is far more suitable than a medical training. It is in the nature of nurse-training to follow orders and this is what clinical guidelines appear to be about.

The training of doctors on the other hand is to do with being able to 'think outside the box' as it were. Doctors are required to assemble facts to do with a patient's problem in order to make a diagnosis which is indeed assembling these facts into a 'box'. They also need to use their judgement in following rules when managing patients. In consequence they are uneasy with having to follow guidelines in the obedient way that nurses do.

The nurse's knowledge of the guidelines is therefore likely to be better than that of the doctor with resulting conflict. Often the doctor will then leave the nurse to look after guideline-managed diseases, eg asthma, the results being the de-skilling of the doctor as he/she is no longer sees that type of patient. The consequence of that is the patient is then without the medical expertise which can still be needed from time to time. The result here is 'dumbed down clinical care'.

There are numerous other unforeseen consequences that result from the Nursing Profession seeking to raise its status. The nursing leaders in the 1990s moved nurse training to degree level as a consequence of their thinking that caring was demeaning to women in the context of the 'handmaiden' idea. This unravelled when these nurses eventually came to look after patients. These nurses then discovered that patients required care and not the application of the 'science' taught them in college. Furthermore the doctors had had a more scientific training than they had.Not surprisingly this is disillusioning and morale sapping for the nurses.

Medico-legally too nurses as separate health care professionals have become more vulnerable in comparison to when they were working more closely with the doctors. In those days in the easy to and fro between doctors and nurses on the wards and in the absence of a 'them and us' situation, problems and difficulties were easier to sort out. Because of this increase in vulnerability of nurses, the Nursing Profession has become more defensive as well as becoming more institutionalised.The consequence are more rules and regulations as to what nurses can and cannot do. There has been a proliferation of 'dismissible offences' for nurses, -again hardly morale boosting!

Despite or perhaps because of all this, most of the complaints from patients nowadays are about nurses. Job satisfaction amongst the nurses is poor leading to poor retention of nurses, shortage of nurses hence the huge expense of agency nurses. Agency nurses can not be as effective as the permanent nurses who know the patients and the way about their hospital.

A further consequence is the 'promotion' as they and the NHS see it, of clinical nurses to be managers.

There is of course also a higher salary for a manager than there is for a nurse. The consequences here are twofold:the loss of a clinical nurse and yet another manager who has been trained not to co-operate with doctors.

There are of course many more reasons why the job of being a nurse in the UK is so unsatisfactory. They spend far too much time on paperwork and form filling than dealing with patients. Go to any ward and the nurses are gathered around the desk dealing with their forms and talking to each other rather than talking to the patients which is what previous generations of nurses spent their time doing.

Another factor is that the 'brownie points' in the organisation are more numerous outside the wards than on the wards hence the perceived importance of the forms by which assessments are made of how well a ward is functioning. In terms of the need for the care of the patients on the ward, this appears to be back to front, and unfortunately typical of much of what is going on in the NHS today.

In summary, to me what has happened to the Nursing Profession with direct effect on the NHS over the decades is a tragedy.

Nurses of previous generations now in their senior years are in agreement. When these retired nurses need nursing care, they are often upset at what has happened to their profession now that they are at the patient end of the NHS.

In the early decades of the NHS the British Nurse was really excellent. unfortunately the 'doctor's handmaiden' notion then threw a spanner into the works.

I was reminded how good these nurses in the 60s and 70s were when a cohort of Philippine nurses arrived on our wards a few years ago. These nurses from the Philippines were caring, competent, knowledgeable, loved by the patients and were a relief for the doctors to work with.

There has to be a way back.

## Chapter Five

## Guidelines and their consequences

Advances in medical treatment since my medical school days have been enormous, resulting in diseases becoming much more treatable. If the treatment that is available is given to all UK patients, disease outcomes in this country would be as good if not better than in other Western Countries. Unfortunately so far as many disease outcomes are concerned,the UK is way down the Western Countries league tables. The medical care in this country is patchy and very uneven despite being delivered largely within a single health system.

As an aside, those who believe that the days are numbered for the NHS will question the word 'despite' and change it to a 'because'.

Understandably therefore attempts have been made by the Department of Health to improve the standards of health care across the country and in addition to have treatment underpinned by a solid evidence base.One of these measures is the institution of guidelines through the National Institution of Clinical Excellence (NICE)

There will be a section on the fairly new and fashionable term 'evidence base' in chapter ten,and from the meaning of the words, guidelines arising should be good and sound.The question is how soundly based is the evidence in every case.

In my own speciality of chest medicine, evidence is produced by clinical trials of the drugs in question. When one finds out however that in the very common Chronic Obstructive Pulmonary Disease(COPD) which kills 25,000 people in the UK every year, only 10% of patients with this disease are eligible for entry into these trials, one has to question their validity and therefore the evidence base that then results in the COPD guidelines.

Leaving that aside, under the meaning of the word 'guideline' there shouldn't then be any problem.Clinical freedom should be preserved as they only 'guide'. The reality on the ground however is very different

For the expert the guidelines are of course irrelevant with their own patients. They recognise the heterogeneity of diseases, their fuzzy boundaries and are also permitted to assess patient variables and to use their clinical judgement.

Not surprisingly their practice is often at variance with the guidelines and incidentally can be cheaper as they are of course allowed discretion to tailor treatment according to how the patient responds.

The expertise of everyone else treating patients is very variable. The less the expertise of course, the less relevant will be the word 'guide'.Given that non-adherence to guidelines can be questioned by any number of people in the system, eg pharmacists, managers, finance directors etc as well as by patients, life is too short and work pressure too great for most doctors to deviate from the so-called 'guidelines'. Medico legally as well, the doctor feels safer following the guidelines.

Looking forward over the years there is a distinct risk that this dominance of guidelines over how doctors treat patients will end up with dumbed-down medicine delivered by dumbed-down doctors who will no longer need to know the rationale behind what is in the guidelines! In his 2003 book,'Hippocratic Oaths' Raymond Tallis states that,- 'medicine may become the first blue-collar profession,delivered by supine,sessional functionaries'.(See the section in chapter 10 on algorithms and the downsides of an 'algorithm' culture).

At the moment though the one group of health care workers who like and get on with guidelines are nurses.Doctors on the other hand have difficulties with guidelines.It is in the nature of nurse-training to follow orders and this in a sense is what clinical guidelines appear to be about.

The training of doctors on the other hand is different.They are required to assemble clinical data in order to make a diagnosis. Clinical judgement and clinical acumen are attributes by which a doctor is judged by his/her colleagues. By their very nature and training therefore doctors will be uneasy with having to follow guidelines in the obedient way that nurses do.

Given all of this, the nurse's knowledge of the guidelines is likely to be better than that of the doctor. This state of affairs can and does result in conflict. Often the doctor will then leave the nurse to look after guideline-managed diseases, eg asthma, the results being the de-skilling of the doctor as he/she is no longer seeing that type of patient. Another consequence is for the patient, and it is the absence of medical expertise and authority when the guideline advice should be ignored or improved upon.The result: 'dumbed down clinical care'

Guidelines allow algorithms of clinical care which can be costed and controlled by management.However the doctor sees the doctor-patient relationship as central to medical care and clinical freedom as essential.In consequence control by managers, however indirect is inevitably seen as being to the detriment of patient care.

The unforeseen consequences of the provision of guidelines many of which are negative, pose a number of interesting questions.In my own speciality of respiratory medicine there are big problems resulting from the guidelines in that they cause much confusion among patients, GPs, non-respiratory consultants and this is to do with diagnostic labels that need to be attached to patients for them to gain entry into guideline management of their respiratory problem. Therefore patients who haven't been labelled as being asthmatic, but could respond to anti-asthmatic treatment in for instance the treatment of a cough, are likely to be denied that treatment precisely because they 'don't have asthma'. In addition guideline-managed diseases are so heterogenous that attaching a diagnosis to an actual patient is rather more difficult, (at times it should actually be impossible) than realised by the writers of the guidelines.Similar situations may very well exist in other specialities.

Leaving this specialised aspect of guidelines aside, would the introduction of guidelines in the early decades of the NHS have created the problems that they have caused more recently? The doctors of those times would  have considered that question as silly given that a competent doctor would have been expected to know their contents already.A check list or pocket text book would have sufficed. (Nowadays we have in addition the iPhone!). Rather than guidelines, if they wanted nurse-involvement to manage patients they would have issued written instructions. Certainly they would have retained responsibility over patient care.

Coming to more recent times, were doctors asked whether and why guidelines should be introduced? I have no memories of such a question and had I and my colleagues been asked, our answer would have been the same as our predecessors. Arguments such as medicine is now more complex, wouldn't have altered the response.

A view is possible that it is the generators of the guidelines, the 'experts' who have overcomplicated and disturbed the clinical management of patients.They are often in receipt of all kinds of benefits, directly and indirectly from the pharmaceuticals and have their authority in virtue of their position on NICE guideline committees  This whole system has the power as outlined above which causes the negative aspects of guidelines as detailed here, the most important of which is the undermining of doctors with loss of their job satisfaction, as they can no longer look after patients professionally as they used to be able to do.

The question remains, what is the use of national guidelines for treating patients in an NHS where this should be the responsibility of well trained, up to date and competent doctors who shouldn't in fact need these guidelines and certainly shouldn't have to be bothered by them?

**Chapter Six**

**Lung function tests and chest medicine**

Within the actual practice of medicine itself there are examples of unforeseen  consequences which have resulted from changes in disease management.

Within my own speciality patients referred to me frequently complain of health care workers giving contradictory advice and information. GPs also complain of the confusions surrounding the management of their patients with the two commonest diseases of the chest which are asthma and chronic obstructive pulmonary disease (COPD) and in consequence have for the most part handed the management of these patients to their nurses to be guideline-managed.GPs themselves don't like, understand or get on with guidelines. This leads not only to the de-skilling of doctors but also to a reduction in standards of medical care, in effect a 'dumbing down' in relation to these diseases. (see the last chapter,-'Guidelines and their consequences').To cap it all, chest specialists complain about the incompetence of GPs in dealing with these diseases.

All of these problems can be seen as a result of certain developments in chest medicine, mostly to do with nomenclature and classification. Much of this originates from the undue importance attached to lung function tests.In a scientific age objective data such as numbers matter, unduly at times. Numbers are what respiratory physiologists provide!In addition their science in its further reaches is rather too difficult for most to understand and therefore tends not to be questioned.In consequence of both of these facts, it is not surprising, also from a sociological point of view, that lung function test results have had such a dominant role in chest medicine.This is unfortunate from at least two points of view.

Firstly it over complicates as well as gets in the way of the management of the common and serious diseases, asthma and COPD.

Secondly it ignores the usefulness of taking as much notice of their symptoms in the assessment and management of these patient as on their lung function test results.

Inflammation of the airways is the cause of the common and serious chest diseases, asthma and COPD.Inflammation can produce abnormal lung function tests.It can also bring about symptoms, of coughing, wheezing, shortness of breath, chest pain/discomfort and the production of sputum.These symptoms occur in various combinations or in isolation. They are not necessarily always accompanied by a reduction in measurable lung function. However as symptoms don't have the objective status provided by lung function tests, the latter will have more notice taken of them by medical science and importantly, in designing clinical trials of possible treatments. These clinical trials result in an evidence base which then underpins and gives authority to the resulting guidelines.

To some the evidence base in respiratory medicine needs examination.It is extraordinary that in the major controlled clinical trials in COPD, only 10% of patients with these disease were eligible for these trials!

The lung function test of which most notice is taken in asthma and COPD is the volume of air that the patient can blow out in one second. This is known as the FEV1(forced expiratory volume in one second)As the airways become narrower as a result of inflammation, the FEV1 result will worsen and improve with effective treatment As the bronchi narrow and less airflow is possible, the patient at some point will feel breathless. Given this, one would expect that there would be a correspondence between the degree of breathlessness and changes in FEV1.Surprisingly this is not always the case. As an example the degree of breathlessness in COPD is not as closely related to the FEV1 loss as one might have expected. This is also true in asthma.The reason for this discordance between airway calibre loss as measured by the FEV1 and the sensation of breathlessness, one of the symptoms mentioned above, is that inflammation of the airways per se can cause a feeling of breathlessness.

Inflammation of the airways as in asthma can cause the production of large quantities of phlegm rather than very significant drops in FEV1. This can result in the patient's asthma not being diagnosed and treated correctly.Google"excessive mucus, shortness of breath", and you will find numerous personal stories from sufferers, coupled with accounts of unsatisfactory medical consultations in which asthma as a possibility doesn't get a mention.In my experience these patients can respond well to anti-asthma treatment

There are many other examples that also show that lung function test results have to be taken in conjunction with patient symptoms as parameters for assessing patient management. As it is, doing lung function tests in a patient with a cough is often a waste of time.The liability to cough can prevent adequate effort on the part of the patient and this will of course result in a spuriously low result.

One of the problems of introducing symptoms as an assessment tool is that an evidence base is required to underpin the validity of the notion that symptoms can act as disease markers and can also be a means of measuring treatment responses.

There are a number of breath tests that indicate bronchial inflammation. Correlating these with the presence of symptoms and their response to treatment would be important.Bronchial reactivity which is measurable, increases with bronchial inflammation and can be measured and similarly correlated with symptoms. Medical students, trainee GPs and trainee hospital doctors are always in search of interesting projects and these if appropriately supervised will deliver an adequate evidence base.This could be established rapidly.

A positive consequence of this interest in symptoms, after all they are what actually bother the patient, will of course be that more attention will be paid to that individual in distinction to attending only to their test results!

Having established an evidence base, symptoms could then go into the mix for patient assessment and treatment.The question then would be, is the precision, effort and training which is required at the moment to carry out lung function testing still necessary? As it happens lung function testing can also be very stressful for patients. Technicians who do a variety of other tests on patients, report that getting patients to breathe out forcefully as is required, is by far the most stressful test they carry out. Patients can even fall over(they need to sit)and faint doing them.

As an alternative, a simple cheap handheld spirometer can be used to deliver a repeatable and satisfactory FEV1, not stressful to the patient. This inexpensive apparatus is available for any GP to buy.

For GPs the currency as it were with which they interact with patients are of course symptoms. With this new significance of symptoms in managing patients with asthma and COPD, and with the use of the readily available cheap ways of measuring the FEV1, the GP could be back in charge of managing these patients with the help of the nurses.

The range of drugs available to treat these patients are well within the capability of a GP to learn and when the management of these patients is un-coupled from national guidelines (see chapter on guidelines) doctors would again feel professionally competent to deal with these patients.

Coming back to  difficulties to do with nomenclature and classification, the problems to do with the names given as diagnoses to patients are numerous and not just in my speciality but across the whole of medical practice.

In respiratory medicine, 'asthma' as a diagnosis is handed out far too frequently to patients.People are naturally frightened having a disease which can be fatal and whose common sense meaning is well known and more often as not doesn't tally with what the patient is experiencing!

Nowadays anyone who responds to anti-asthma treatment is liable to be told they have asthma.Ironically anti-asthma treatment, which would be effective in some patients is frequently withheld because 'you don't have asthma'!

Those who are told they have 'COPD', Google it and in the majority of cases are falsely informed that they have a progressive fatal disease!

A paradigmatic shift in the nomenclature used in dealing with the common inflammatory conditions of the airways is required.In the meantime sticking to the basics of what is going on as outlined here will be helpful to patients as well as those looking after them.

Finally and at least as important as anything here is applying the basics as outlined to reducing the use of antibiotics in primary care.The commonest unnecessary use of antibiotics is in so-called 'chest infections' which in fact are usually episodes of airway inflammation triggered by viruses.

The consequences of the proposals in this chapter should be that the problems at the top of this chapter would no longer exist.

In addition the cost of looking after these patients should be less and more importantly, their care much improved.

**Chapter Seven**

**Specialisation and the loss of the Generalist**

I was appointed as a Consultant Physician in general medicine with a special interest in respiratory medicine to a District General Hospital in 1977. The role of the General Physician in the hospital was to be competent in dealing with all the non-surgical diseases occurring in the local population which the General Practitioners needed help with, either as outpatients or inpatients.In addition if the surgeons in the hospital were puzzled by patients under their care, they would ask the General Physician for help. Their expression was that they needed one of the 'clever' doctors to sort things out.

The General Physician consultant has disappeared from UK medical practice and replaced by specialist consultants.

The specialist consultants may no longer feel competent to deal with patients whose problem lies outside their speciality. Hence the patient is referred to another specialist. One of the results is the fragmentation of patient care in secondary care.No one individual such as the Consultant General Physician of former times is in overall charge of all aspects of the care of the patient.Medicine has become more complex over the years but the question is whether in terms of best patient care the degree of specialisation has become excessive, and the loss of the General Physician a real loss to patient care.

In primary care too in relation to my own speciality (see lung function tests and chest medicine ) one of the results of over-specialisation and the inevitable guidelines (see chapter on guidelines) has been the de-skilling of the General Practitioner in dealing with the very common respiratory conditions in their patients.

Another personal experience prompts the question of over-specialisation. The consultant General Physician as was also dealt with most of the common endocrine problems in the local population Some years after my appointment I persuaded a top endocrine specialist to do a monthly clinic in our hospital. After a year or two it was decided to discontinue the clinic as my General Physician colleagues and I were not referring a sufficient number of patients to the endocrine clinic to make it worthwhile to continue with. Ironically not long after, we appointed two specialist endocrine consultants prompted by the fact that the diabetic clinic was becoming overwhelmed with the number of patients. For my own interest I went to one of their clinical meetings a year or two later and had great difficulty in following the technical discussions taking place. My difficulty in understanding discussions about patients who in the absence of our new endocrine consultants I and my General Physician colleagues would have been looking after suggests two possibilities.

The first possibility is that these patients had been looked after inadequately by the general Physicians prior to the arrival of specialist endocrinologists.

The second possibility is that as all groups of individuals do, endocrinologists have developed their own 'endocrine speak' and practice but were not necessarily treating the patients much better than they had been by the generalist.

From my own observations within my speciality, the generalist and this includes particularly the GP, can in my opinion be trusted to deal adequately with the majority of patients.

Debate which I hope this publication will result in, is needed.

# Chapter Eight

## Gender and medical school entry

When I went to medical school in 1960, out of the 50 students in my year, less than ten were female.There are medical schools now where up to 70% are female. This is the result of a medical degree being highly sought after, and because the entry criteria are much about A levels.Females at 18 are better at A levels than males, hence the gender difference in the medical schools.

In my years as a doctor I have not found women doctors any better than their male counterparts which brings into question the female preponderance in medical schools the result of which is more female doctors than male.For many of these female doctors a part time career will be their choice, certainly when they are younger with children and families. This is very much less likely for male doctors. The tax payer supports the training of doctors to the tune of £500,000 for each doctor and appear to be unaware that they are likely to get less doctoring for their money from a newly qualified female doctor than from a male doctor.

A public debate is needed about medical school entry. There are a number of fair ways of increasing the proportion of males in medical schools but the politicians both medical and non-medical would need a lot more courage than they seem capable of in our age of political correctness. There are though more consequences to the increasing proportion of female doctors to consider.

Doctor-Patient relationships in important ways, are about continuity of care where the doctor knows the patient and in consequence the patient trusts that doctor. The medicine practised in these circumstances is likely to be better, more efficient and less costly. The common complaint in the UK in General Practice is, 'I never see the same doctor twice'. There are other reasons in play, which I will deal with in other parts of this publication, but the disappearance of the full-time GP, with a list of patients that the GP knows and is personally responsible for, is incompatible with more and more part-time doctors replacing the full-time doctor of previous times.

As an aside a consequence of the disappearance of the so-called old-fashioned GP is that those that can afford it now pay for their own private GP. Needless to say, private General Practice is now flourishing in the UK, often providing high class doctoring, delivered by enthusiastic doctors who see themselves as having escaped the deadening and depressing climate that had existed for them in the NHS. They are grateful to be able to practise the medicine that they were trained for.Ironically these practices could be used as models at some future date for re-discovering NHS General Practice as it used to be.

Apparently now forgotten is that in years gone by, General Practice was seen by the rest of the world as the 'jewel in the crown' of the NHS. This is increasingly less so.In the last 50 years there have of course been many other changes in society and these have also had an influence in the NHS.Ideas to do with 'work-life balance', gender equality, social equality, patient as customer/client etc, all valuable in their own way, have over the years all had an influence on an organisation as large and complex as the NHS.

In my generation medicine could and often did take over the lives of doctors, often to the benefit of patients, but not infrequently to the detriment of the doctor. New ways of looking at a doctor's life and at the needs of patients were necessary. What has however been ignored over the decades in the NHS is that there is always a mix of values in competition in any organisation, each if pursued without adequate consideration to others can result in negative consequences, often unforeseen.

It is those multiple unforeseen negative consequences that have made the NHS increasingly less workable and what this publication is about.

**Chapter Nine**

**Shipman and the 'Shipman effect'**

Harold Frederick Shipman, (14 January 1946 – 13 January 2004) was a British doctor and one of the most prolific serial killers in recorded history. Although Shipman is the only British doctor who has been found guilty of murdering his patients, the fact that a doctor was able to kill repeatedly, possibly 250 victims, and not be found out doing so over a number of years, resulted in the review and modification of much of Britain's legal structure concerning health care, death certification and medicine. More significant though was the resulting cultural change in relation to medicine.

Once the notion of the need to safeguard and monitor the decisions made by doctors is voiced, much of what a doctor is about comes into question. Although science and objective facts underpin medical decision making, an important ingredient to medical practice is known as the 'art of medicine'.

The ingredients to the 'art of medicine' are a mixture of intuition, experience, clinical acumen, wider education, wisdom etc. These are all rather nebulous and the computer world has justifiably brought much of this under scrutiny, but at the end of the day some gardeners have 'green fingers' as do some doctors. In other words some doctors are better than others and not necessarily for any identifiable reasons.

'Clinical judgement' and 'clinical freedom' are seen by the medical profession as essential to practising medicine, that is to being a doctor. Medicine is a discipline where clinical decisions have to be made even when the circumstances are uncertain. Treatment cannot always wait for a definitive diagnosis to be made and in any case definitive diagnoses are not always possible.In these circumstances, the doctor then falls back on having to use his/her clinical judgement. This in part is what is known as 'clinical freedom'. Clinical freedom however is practised with the knowledge that any judgement made has to be open to scrutiny at the time or subsequently. Doctors who find it too difficult to make clinical decisions in uncertain clinical situations will if sensible, and if this is possible for them, move into non-clinical areas of medicine of which there are many. Most doctors however remain in clinical medicine.

As the Shipman case unravelled and for a considerable time after, I can remember as a recurring theme colleagues reacting to the consequent so-called 'safe guarding' changes. To us many of these were seen as inconveniences, even as insults.

-' Shipman is mad but we are not'.
-'What possible reason could he have had'.
-'My name isn't Harold Shipman, why on earth do we have to do that?'
-'This is all because of Shipman'.
-And so on.

Since Shipman, but of course not entirely because of Shipman, there has developed an increasing need for doctors to be able to justify their clinical decisions. This is no bad thing but needless to say there are negative consequences.

-'Covering your backside' is time consuming and can get in the way of looking after patients.

-'If it hasn't been written down it hasn't happened'. This is a recurring proposition when patient notes are examined in for example dealing with a patient complaint or a medico legal case. In a court of law of course, this statement will carry a lot of weight. The proposition presupposes though that everything important in patient care can be written down. This isn't true in ordinary life, neither is it true in clinical medicine. The apparent need though to record 'everything' will certainly result in much more paperwork.

If this extra paperwork was entirely in the narrative that would be one thing and more likely to correspond to what has actually happened. This is in distinction to the endless forms and tick boxes that now plague the modern health care professional. The forms and tick boxes require the prior systemisation of clinical situations. This isn't always possible as clinical situations are not all stereotyped and in consequence this systemisation and classification will at times be spurious and be unable to capture what does happen. In addition and inevitably the forms will dictate to some extent what the clinician does. This can hamper how the clinician performs and in addition lead to clinical mistakes.

Finally some of the frustrations of form filling is explicable on the basis of the not infrequent mismatches between the reality that is presupposed by the designers of forms and the reality of an actual clinical situation. These mismatches if un-noticed can also lead to mistakes in patient care.

Tick boxes etc do have other origins of course than Shipman. For example, a direct consequence of the internal market, the purchaser-provider split of health care introduced in the 80s, (see chapter ten), is the need to itemise what is being 'bought and sold'. The 'invoicing of health care' inevitably has as consequence forms and tick boxes.

Coming back to the Shipman effect, there has been a dramatic reduction in the number of single-handed GPs.In the ten years 2002 to 2012, the number of single handed GPs went down by 42%Though there are other explanations for this, Shipman was indeed working on his own.The Shipman Report did not directly recommend this reduction, it did state though that there was not enough safeguarding and monitoring of doctors' decisions in single -handed general practice.

The reduction in the number of single-handed practices is a shame as it was always my impression that many of the really good GPs in the catchment area of the hospital where I worked were in fact single-handed. My explanation for this was that these doctors had taken on the continuing and therefore full responsibility of the care of their patients.

Taking full and continuing responsibility for patients is from many points of view beneficial to patients.It has become a rarity in the NHS, certainly in the cities, and for the most part now is only to be obtained in private practice. Whitehall as well as the medical establishment no longer like GPs working on their own and in recent years it is the single handed GPs who I have seen finding themselves in trouble with the increasing bureaucracy of the NHS. There are all sorts of ways of course for the bureaucrats who run the NHS to put pressure on doctors that they disapprove of and these will include single-handed GPs!

Undoubtedly the negative aspects of the Shipman effect would have been less in previous years when much of what happened in the NHS was still being dictated by doctors .Unfortunately Shipman occurred when increasingly doctors were no longer being listened to. The 'age of management' in the NHS had arrived and managers rather than doctors were responsible for much of the 'Shipman Effect'.

Unfortunately the leaders of the medical profession did not look closely enough at the negative consequences of the reactions to the shock of what Shipman had done and been permitted to do by the system. The mistake was not to listen to the clinicians looking after patients in the aftermath of Shipman.

What was obvious though was that the public needed reassurance about their doctors and the medical profession generally. As it happened though there was already a perception amongst doctors for the need for more openness and transparency in their dealings with their patients.Doctors if still being listened to would, as a result of Shipman, have accelerated this, but the extra forms, tick boxes and restrictions generated in the NHS as part of the Shipman Effect would be unlikely to have occurred to bother doctors as they have done.

Bothering doctors is bad for doctors as well as bad for patient care!

**Chapter Ten**

**Ideas, fashions, notions, aphorisms, concepts, occurrences etc and the NHS debate**

Debate and the NHS was there at the beginning. A large part of the medical profession was dragged kicking and screaming into it in 1948 but like the rest of the country has for the most part been emotionally attached to it over the years. Unfortunately the reality is that many doctors are now unhappy working in the NHS and cannot see it surviving as it is.They find it dysfunctional and frustrating. Much gets in the way of what they have been trained to do.One of the intentions of this publication is to start a conversation about the NHS.

I have already picked out and detailed various topics to highlight reasons why the NHS is in trouble. More could have been analysed  but that task could have been endless and the sooner the conversation starts around the need for a different approach for the NHS, the better.

This section of part two will consist of a list, some with short notes, of items which at different times have been relevant.Others are still current.

Here goes:

1)Not a penny of the tax payers' money is to be wasted'

-How much money has been spent attempting to realise this promise? How much frustration and poorer patient care has been, and is still being generated by it? What is the problem with trusting the highly trained and still idealistic NHS work force which is actually involved in patient care?

2)The internal market, -splitting the activities in the NHS into provider and purchaser ones.

-The notion of Adam Smith's 'invisible hand' as an alternative to top-down government was fashionable in the 80s and led to the idea of introducing competition between purchasers and providers in the NHS. This was seen as a means of improving the NHS.Innovative GPs did indeed improve their patients' care but unfortunately their success undermined the basic idea of the NHS of having to be equal up and down the land.

As time has gone on, the purchaser/provider exercise has proved of questionable value as well as costly and clumsy. It has been and still is causing difficulties in managing patients across the different parts of the NHS especially between the GPs and hospitals.

So far as Adam Smith is concerned, his 'invisible hand' also needed in the mix 'moral sentiments' as in his other book. For these to work however, individuals need to matter as they used to 50 years ago. This is no longer the case.For 'moral sentiments' to be relevant in a system, the individuals in it have as a matter of logical necessity to matter.

3)Evidence-based medical practice

- Archie Cochrane (1909-1988) a doctor and epidemiologist was correct in stating that evidence as demonstrated in randomised clinical trials is needed to underpin how patients should be treated.Unfortunately like most good ideas the term 'evidence based' has tended to become a mantra.As already pointed out this notion needs constant scrutiny.(see chapter five)

4)Shift work for junior doctors was introduced in 1991.

-Although there were good reasons at the time for reviewing how junior doctors worked, the instinctive reaction of more experienced doctors was that a professional's work should be open ended and that shifts were therefore wrong. The consequences of introducing shifts for juniors, many unforeseen and negative, are numerous. Leaving aside the junior hospital doctors' strike of 2016, the important casualties include the poorer training and experience available for the juniors and the destruction of the clinical 'firms' which worked well for doctors and their patients. Interestingly and reassuring is how much the juniors ignore dictates to do with shifts when they see what is necessary for a particular patient's safety.However, and inevitably, continuity of patient care and other examples of good practice possible before 1991 suffered.The idea of 'now being off duty' although relevant to work-life balance, does have downsides. These also need balancing.

5)An insurance system to replace our single-payer health system, the NHS

-The USA is thinking of moving in the opposite direction precisely because of their experiences within their insurance-dominated health service. They would be well advised to take note of the problems we have allowed to happen as detailed in this publication, and then look at our future attempts to make the NHS become successful again. My suggestion for achieving the latter is in Part Three.

6)Risk management.

-So much of modern life is about risk and its management. Frequently this results in large expenditures of money and effort the need for which is often poorly examined. In medicine this has resulted in a significant shift into managing the risk of diseases occurring.This needs constant scrutiny particularly as risk factors tend to morph into full-blown diseases with all sorts of unforeseen consequences in dealing with these 'diseases'.

7)Process v patient care

-Doctors readily agree that too much of their work is to do with observing 'process' rather than directly related to dealing with patients.This wasn't always so.

There are many reasons for this, albeit some to the benefit of patients safety.

A major reason is however to do with accountability. This has shifted from the simple and straight forward accountability which is intrinsic to individuals relating to each other as described in chapter one.In today's NHS, accountability is supposed to be deliverable by the 'processes' put in place by multi-disciplinary and national committees and The Department Of Health.This 'accountability' is impersonal and in consequence artificial and unsatisfactory in comparison to how it was.An example is how complaints are dealt with.This process,as it tends to be impersonal,is often lengthy and not infrequently doesn't really provide satisfaction for the complainant.

8) Medico-legal, Tabloid and 'covering-your-back' issues.

-These are responsible for much of the 'process' as in 7) and is costly to the NHS.Again much of this can be dealt with by individuals taking personal responsibility.As an example, a complaint about the care of a patient should be the responsibility of the consultant concerned rather than how it is dealt with nowadays,- by the complaints department

From a wider perspective and given that the NHS is to do with the common good, Parliament and appropriate legislation is required.'Ambulance chasers' and lawyers need to be discouraged.Health care professionals need more looking after.'Playing it safe' isn't always to the benefit of patients.

Finally earlier settlements of complaints as are likely with the consultants dealing with them, are likely to be less expensive and less traumatic to all concerned.

9)Algorithmic patient care eg the Liverpool Care Pathway.

-Predictably the latter as a way of dealing with patients at the end of their lives was abandoned.The former also needs constant scrutiny. An algorithmic culture should worry us.

10)Loss of local medical societies some of which had been in existence, often for more than 100 years.

-Hospital doctors and General Practitioners no longer know each other.They used to and that certainly helped in the care of their patients.

11)District general hospitals morphing into trusts.

-This was to do with internal market vocabulary. This new way of looking at local hospitals allows their survival to be threatened.

12)Medical Ethics.

-The mistake is to think that this fairly recent industry gives answers to what to do in ethically difficult situations. Ideally the experts in medical ethics should do no more than analyse the circumstances in an ethical framework.In my experience intuition still rules and if well informed, should.

13)Health and safety.

-This has done a lot of good over the years but when uttered in innumerable situations, 'Health and Safety', has become a way that seems to be intended to stop people doing the obvious. This does however lend itself to a culture that has developed in the NHS since management took over.

The question is what will happen to 'health and safety' following the radical re-think of the NHS which I am proposing

14)Conveyor belt of care.

-The idea suggested here is as impersonal as the concepts by which health strategists/academics appear to look at the NHS.

15)The Ten minute GP consultation.

-This has arisen in recent years from various circumstances in General Practice.Ten minutes is now stipulated as the period of time a patient needs to have a problem sorted out by the GP. This idea would have shocked previous generations of GPs!

16)Clinical Coding.

-Clinical Coding as defined is 'the translation of medical terminology as written by the clinician to describe a patient's complaint, problem, diagnosis, treatment or reason for seeking medical attention, into a coded format' which is nationally and internationally recognised. Amazingly in hospitals, when this coded format is decoded into language, it bears only a poor resemblance to how doctors actually communicate with each other about their patients.

For obvious reasons this matters in many ways. Funding in both the NHS and in medical insurance is dependant on accurate coding. How can that be possible where the language used in clinical care is at variance with Clinical-Coding language? Inevitably too doctors and their teams are unable to take much part in clinical coding as they do not understand it and therefore find it difficult to take part in what the system attaches so much importance and funding to. This is yet another example of a mismatch between on-the-ground patient-care reality, and what the systems, the NHS in the UK and medical insurance industry in the USA operate by.

I suspect that a lot of this complexity and incomprehensibility is the accidental consequence of the endless arguments that must have occurred over the years between insurance companies and medics.This accident needs to be sorted out in order for doctors and coding departments to be able to talk sensibly to each other.

17)The Medical Personnel Department becomes The Human Resources Department in the mid-80s

-Individuals are now liable to be seen as a resource-part in the system.

18)Every plane crash reduces the risk of flying.

-Would that were true in the NHS

19)Institutions do not have a sense of honour.People do!
-Individuals working in the NHS need to matter again. They used to.

## Chapter Eleven

## The apprentice system and the medical profession

Medicine has always fascinated me and continues to do so. The same was true for many of my contemporaries. When we met colleagues for example in the corridor, the doctors' car park or in the doctors' dining room (now both gone), the topic of conversation would often be about patients either because they presented an interesting problem or for advice. This is no longer the case.Now the topic of conversation with a colleague is too often about the hassle working in the NHS. What appears to be absent now is the fascination and the enthusiasm in medicine that used to exist.This chapter is about the effect of the loss of a type of training in Britain and the effect that this has had on the medical profession in this country.

I and my contemporaries had what is now derided by educationalists as an 'apprentice-type' medical eduction.Educationalists worry me. The College of Police have just said that policemen require degrees to do their jobs adequately and I note that the bobby is being withdrawn from patrolling the street,'the beat'.The Royal College of Nursing went down this road  25 years ago. Nursing degrees happened and the consequences, unforeseen by the nursing profession, but not by the doctors, were at the very least, disappointing (see chapter four).

There is a saying, 'if you can't do it, teach it; if you can't teach, teach teachers'. I would add to that, 'if you can't or don't want to do any of that and are interested in education, there are well paid job-opportunities as an educationalist'. The problem is that when 'learning' is dissected, analysed and researched by academics as happens in the discipline of Education, and when this is all taken up by educationalists, much of what it is to be a policeman, nurse or doctor has not been looked at.In addition much is introduced into curricula for theoretical and even evidence-based reasons that actually gets in the way of what is needed to carry out these jobs.

From my own experience of being in charge of training and education in my hospital over a period of 20 years, I used to attend regular regional meetings over that period to do with 'developing' training and education for junior doctors, and increasingly I was concerned that things were going in the wrong direction.

They were!

At this point it is worth recapping my own so-called 'apprentice-type' training. When I moved on to the wards as a medical student I had acquired a comprehensive grounding in the basic medical sciences and what then interested me was finding out what had gone wrong with the patient in terms of my understanding of that scientific knowledge.

I was taught in what is now known as an 'apprentice-type' way, that is learning from the doctors of all seniorities in the team managing the patients.During my three years of clinical training as a medical student I had no tests, examinations or formal assessments at any time.This is in stark contrast to the modern medical students who absent themselves from clinical teaching and ward rounds in order to study in the library for forthcoming tests!

In my day the doctors on the team or firm, would make sure that the students were up to speed with what was going on with the patients and how that related to basic medical sciences, pathology and therapy. There were of course final examinations in order to qualify as a doctor. Failures were unusual.

This 'apprentice-type' training continued until I became a consultant by my taking note of how the 'apprentice master', the consultant in whose team I was working , dealt with the patients and with the discussions within the successive consultant-led teams of which I was an increasingly senior member. All of this was of course supplemented by lectures, seminars and reading.Clinical meetings where clinical cases in the hospital were discussed by all the consultants in the hospital and their juniors, was again a form of 'apprentice-type' learning. As a consultant I kept up to date by attending lectures, courses, clinical meetings and reading the medical literature but most importantly training my juniors and also learning from them. In a sense I had become in turn an 'apprentice master'.

What do the educationalists miss in what they call 'apprentice-type' training?For a start the literature on it is far from being comprehensive. The perspective of the 'apprentice' and 'apprentice master' is largely ignored. What was I hoping to achieve during my training both as a medical student and trainee doctor? What am I hoping for in order to remain as a non-trainee doctor by continuing to keep up to date?

The lay public when listening to doctors talking between themselves about what is wrong with a patient, complain that doctors sound as if they are talking 'gobbledegook'. Training to be a doctor has been likened to learning a foreign language. There are of course thousands of new words to be learned but unlike learning a foreign language there are in addition conceptual schemes which are largely to do with what practising medicine is about. None of this 'doctor-speak' is mysterious as it was in previous centuries. All of it can be explained in 'lay-man speak' by doctors when necessary. What we have though is a community, doctors, who when doing their work are not functioning entirely as laypeople do. Being able to function satisfactorily in this community is what it means to be a doctor and that is what learning to be a doctor is about. What happens, and indeed what happens to any apprentice at the end of their training, is the acceptance by their new peers.

By 'apprenticeships' we think more in terms of crafts and trades than professions such as medicine, but belonging to a skilled peer group and what that entails is to a certain extent common across all these groupings. Just as with these other groups, a sense of belonging, maintaining standards, advancing skills and peer pressure is also intrinsic to being a doctor, that is, belonging to the medical profession. Peer pressure amongst doctors is enormous and in consequence doctors tend to be conformist so far as their clinical activities are concerned.

Caution is no bad thing when treating patients. 'That was brave' as a comment on a particular treatment by a doctor is usually seen as a criticism therefore to be known as a 'brave' doctor is probably best avoided. On the upside of this is that the profession can be self policing. On the downside new ideas and treatments can take longer to be adopted than need be. There is of course a further downside such as being too excluding and being seen as such.

Many of the skills that doctors have can in fact be performed with adequate training by non-doctors and the medical profession, if rather reluctantly has accepted the reality of some of that. Not to be forgotten is that what remains unique though to being a doctor, is being able to perform satisfactorily in his/her peer group, the medical profession.

Why is it that the medical profession sees itself as sidelined in the NHS? Why does the medical profession in the UK appear to have had the stuffing knocked out of it? Developments in the NHS in recent years have resulted in doctors feeling that they don't count. Apart from the patient no one else appears to listen to them.It isn't only doctors who see this as being a bad thing.

There are many reasons to explain what has happened over the decades, but central to this is the loss in increasing quantities of the identity and therefore the vigour, assertiveness and authority of the community made up of doctors, the medical profession. The training and education required to join and stay in this peer group is essential to its identity. This identity has been radically undermined with the loss of its 'apprentice/apprentice master' structure.Fundamental to this structure is seeing, doing, being supervised, supervising and conversation up and down this hierarchy of skills in a like-minded community. This is in distinction to accumulating factual knowledge which nowadays appears to need constant testing and this to be conducted in an impersonal way.In a sense an empathic system appears to have been replaced by an autistic one. This has happened gradually over recent years and for the most part, and unfortunately, not noticed by the medical profession.

The pity for the NHS is that it requires a medical profession with its previous authority and standing for it to function efficiently and well. This has been seriously undermined by the loss of the fundamental form of training and education that was had by previous generations of doctors, and which then sustained them, and which I have outlined above.

There are many other reasons why the medical profession in the UK has had its effectiveness diminished.

I will go into these in the next chapter

## Chapter Twelve. The 'Stuff' that has got in the way of the medics and their patients

Motivated doctors are essential for any health service.

How to re-motivate doctors?

Reading US physician comments on Medscape, an international health workers website, the doctors across the Atlantic feel as powerless, frustrated and fed up as their British counterparts. The problem is that on both sides of the Atlantic, 'stuff' has got in the way of practising medicine satisfactorily

This 'stuff' is different in the two systems.

The medical insurance industry in the US has a revenue of $ 730 billion and a workforce of 470, 000. Before they eliminate this complex, costly, inefficient and doctor-debilitating system, if they do, and adopt the single-payer health system, they would be well advised to look at the 'stuff' that has accumulated over the decades in the UK where the NHS has provided most of the health care in Britain since 1948. As a result of continual interference by Central Government and inadequate medical leadership, the 'stuff' in the UK that is now getting in the way of the front-line clinical staff, has made the NHS increasingly unworkable.

The accumulation over the decades of negative unforeseen consequences i.e. 'stuff', is what this publication is about and which has been gone into in some detail in the various sections. Chapter ten also provides some brief notes of other topics, more 'stuff', that ought to be included in the conversation which hopefully this publication will start.

Without this 'stuff' the chances are that we could be back to doctors no longer frustrated at every turn.This will result in well motivated doctors, essential to any health system. This was the case when decades ago the doctors were in a sense in charge of patient care in that they were listened to and responded to by the system. Since then they have been side-lined and are now only listened to by their patients. Except in an emergency i.e.when the 'shit hits the fan' as it were, doctors feel that they are no longer relevant outside their own clinical area even when this is being interfered with by other parts of the organisation.

The reasons for this are many and include the following; the fragmentation of the work force with the build up of seemingly independent bodies of health care professionals where before there were well functioning teams of doctors and nurses;the replacement of administrators by management;the monetisation of so much, for example the purchaser provider split;loss of a hierarchical structure;equity in the sense that everyone's opinion is equal whatever their training and responsibilities etc.

Is there any reason why doctors as a group should not be listened to, responded to and trusted again as used to be the case. With those attitudes to the medics they were in a sense running the NHS. This was so in my early years as a consultant physician? Restoring trust in the clinicians will get rid of much of today's inefficiencies

Forms, documentation and regimentation is the life blood of the current top-down NHS management, implicit is mistrust of the front line clinicians.

Peer pressure, doctor to doctor is enormously powerful, and this coupled with modern information technology will allow transparency to what doctors do and should provide sufficient reassurance to the general public about their health service.

This would replace the expensive and inefficient system that has developed over the years and at present no longer reassures anyone.

So far as the bottom line in today's NHS is concerned, money, there is no need for any change other than the following.

Everything spent money on has to be connected to and seen to be so, to the primary activity in health care and that is a doctor or group of doctors taking responsibility for a patient.

My thesis in this publication is that the basics of medicine need to be returned to in order to 'mend' the NHS.

The base that needs to be returned to is the doctor-patient relationship. The service and money needs to flow from that source. A patient consults a doctor about a problem and that doctor should then be able to take on and discharge that responsibility for the care of that patient with the full support of the service without the thousand and one things involving much manpower and therefore much expense that at the moment stand in the way.

The logistics needed to achieve that have to be worked out.

There shouldn't be any devils in the details.

The expected consequences are a less expensive and much improved NHS.

Undoubtedly there will also be unexpected consequences. Some will be interesting but none are likely to get in the way of patient care.

**Three**

**The way forward**

I do not propose to summarise what I have written as I realise that as a consequence of the inter-connectedness of the many parts of the NHS, there has already been some repetition chapter to chapter.

My proposal for General Practice is as in chapter three and requires a new contract and to repeat, the need to remember the following.

1)General Practice provided the strength of the NHS. Being a family doctor provided the career fulfilment for so many general practitioners in the past.
2)The standards of good medical practice should be regulated by the profession and therefore should not have to be bought by the government as a top-up income (QOF) earned by hitting targets under a performance-related bonus scheme.
3)The GPs need again to be in charge and responsible for their patients 24/7.Years ago, also by cooperating with neighbouring practices, many of them were able to provide this efficiently and well.

As pointed out before, they managed in 2003 to off-load this responsibility for minimal loss of income, The money needed to pay the GPs for resuming this responsibility would be available, firstly by diverting the top-up income(QOF), and secondly a lot of money would be available with the dramatic reduction in A/E and hospital patient numbers that will inevitably follow the GPs again being in charge of their patients.Third, from the money that will no longer be needed to cover off-duty GPs. As it is, this cover excites much negative comment from the public and from the media.

So far as hospitals are concerned the logical conclusion to the contents of this publication is to get back to the situation of 50 years ago when what happened in the NHS was not dominated by the management system that we now have. Doctors were listened to. This should still be the case given their selection, training, experience and the fact that they are actually dealing with the patients. Also in those days those working in the NHS from consultants to ward cleaners mattered as individuals and were able to work together without all the rules and regulations that now get in the way of common sense.

My observations of working in the NHS is that the current power of management is to do with the fact that having the final say about the use of funding dictates what happens. My proposal in the last chapter of part two is that the money should flow from what arises out of the Doctor-patient encounter and be seen to do so. At that point the doctor takes on the responsibility of the care of that patient. Discharging that responsibility has to be fully supported by the hospital. The details of how that is to be carried out and funded needs medical supervision.

To help that line of thought along in what is now such a complicated, complex, cumbersome and unworkable UK health system, the notion of 'zero planning' might help. Here after some catastrophe, delivery of health care has to be started from scratch.Here doctors would be in the frontline of what would happen.

My prescription for the Health Secretary, currently Mr Jeremy Hunt, is as at the front of this book. He ought to ask the medics for their examples of where money is being used in ways that don't help them look after their patients. This would start the conversation that is now needed to restore the NHS to a time when the people on the ground mattered. The doctors need to feel that they are again being listened to, feel that they are again to become responsible for how the NHS functions, and again allowed to feel proud of the nation's health service.

The result should be a more efficient as well as a more human and therefore a more humane NHS for patients and staff.

INDEX

A
Accountability. 63
Adam Smith's invisible hand. 60
             'Moral Sentiments'. 60
Administrators.   9,10,76
A/E   25,79
Age of Management     57
Algorithmic patient care.   34-39,64
          Culture.   34-39,64
Aneurin Bevan.  4,22
Antibiotics,-unnecessary use.   40-46
Apprenticeship Master,      17,68-74
               structure,     68-74
               system,        68-74
               type of education/training  68-74
Art of medicine.47,53
Asthma.   40
Attlee government.     4


B
Back to the future.      12
Basics of patient care.  3,6,9,11,16,17,78
BMA (British Medical Association).19-25

82

Exaggerated egalitarianism   15,16
Expenditure 1, 5.


F
Feelings of nationhood    5,7
Feminism    27
FEV1(forced expiratory volume in one second).   40
Firms 32,35
Fools gold.12
Full-blown diseases.32
Funding.40


G
Gender.    50
Gender equality.   8,52
Generalist.   47-49
General physician.    47-49
'The good days of the NHS'  16
'Gobbledegook'.71
Goodwill   10
Good practice   20
Government mistrust of doctors   9
'Green fingers'.  54
GP(general Practitioner). 3,19-25
GP contract   19-25,79
GP partnership system.  23
Guidelines.  21,27,29,34-39
Guideline-managed diseases.   30,38,40


H
'Handmaidens'.   26-33
Health and Safety.    16,65
Health Care professional.    13-18,26-33,76

Tax payer's money.    14,50,59
Ten minute consultation,      21
Tick boxes.    6,55-6
Tick box tyranny  9
Training-cost for doctors.  50

U
Underfunding      6,10,14
USA.    3,62,75

W
Western Europe  34,5,6,34
Whitehall,-central control.    7,9,12,75
Work-life balance   13,61

Z
Zero planning.    80

26745918R00058

Printed in Great Britain
by Amazon